Rim Amdouni
Elhem Jbebli
Samar Rehayem

# Childhood asthma

Rim Amdouni
Elhem Jbebli
Samar Rehayem

# Childhood asthma

## Care between mother and carer

ScienciaScripts

**Imprint**



Cover image: www.ingimage.com

This book is a translation from the original published under ISBN 978-620-6-71523-8.

Publisher:
Sciencia Scripts
is a trademark of
Dodo Books Indian Ocean Ltd. and OmniScriptum S.R.L publishing group

120 High Road, East Finchley, London, N2 9ED, United Kingdom
Str. Armeneasca 28/1, office 1, Chisinau MD-2012, Republic of Moldova, Europe
Printed at: see last page
**ISBN: 978-620-8-01891-7**

## Table of contents

# INTRODUCTION

Asthma is a heterogeneous, multifactorial disease caused by chronic inflammation of the bronchial tubes. It is characterized by the onset of several paroxysmal or persistent respiratory symptoms, such as dyspnea, dry cough, chest tightness and sibilance. These symptoms are associated with varying degrees of airflow obstruction and hyperresponsiveness of the lower airways [1].

Asthma is the most frequent chronic respiratory pathology in paediatrics, responsible for over 1000 deaths a day worldwide, the majority of which are avoidable. Its prevalence in Tunisia is 10%, with a marked increase in recent decades, making it a real global health problem [2].

Appropriate therapeutic management can help preserve normal lung function and ensure optimal quality of life.

The economic and medical burden of asthma remains high, due to the large number of hospitalizations, and school and work absenteeism for children and their parents. Indeed, hospitalization for asthma attacks or exacerbations remains frequent, especially in the youngest children under 4 years of age [2].

Adherence to treatment in young children depends entirely on their parents. Poor adherence to therapy, as well as incorrect practices (poor inhalation technique, defective hygiene of the inhalation chamber, etc.), are the most common factors leading to hospitalization for asthma attacks or exacerbations [3-4].

This led us to wonder about the reasons for such practices: lack of knowledge on the part of mothers; lack of training on the part of caregivers; other cultural reasons?

To answer these questions, we conducted a cross-sectional CAP study at the Béchir Hamza Children's Hospital. Its objectives were to:

1- Identify factors associated with mothers' knowledge and practices regarding the therapeutic management of asthma in children.
2- Identify factors associated with the knowledge and practices of paramedical caregivers regarding the therapeutic management of asthma in children.

# PATIENTS AND METHODS

## 1. Type and scope of study

We conducted a descriptive observational cross-sectional study aimed at detailing the knowledge, attitudes and practices of mothers and caregivers in the management of asthma in children. The study was carried out at the Béchir Hamza Children's Hospital in Tunis, where it involved the pediatric wards (Pediatrics A, PUC).

Our survey lasted 39 days from 01/02/2024 to 10/03/2023.

## 2. Study population

For the purposes of our work, we recruited two populations: the first made up of mothers and the second made up of caregivers.

### 2.1. Recruiting mothers

- **Inclusion criteria :**
  - Any mother with an asthmatic child under 8 years of age.
  - Consults or has a child admitted between February 1st and March 10 to the Children's Medicine A and CUP departments of the Béchir Hamza Children's Hospital.
- **Criteria for non-inclusion :**

  -Any other family member accompanying the child for consultation or hospitalization (father, grandmother, aunt).
- **Exclusion criteria :**

  -Any mother who refused to participate in the study.

  -Any unfinished questionnaire.

### 2.2. Recruitment of caregivers

- **Inclusion criteria**

- Any pediatric physiotherapist, nurse or technician.
- Working in one of the above-mentioned departments of the Béchir Hamza children's hospital in Tunis.
- Present on the day of our visit

- **Non-inclusion criteria**

- We excluded the other categories of paramedical caregivers, as their knowledge is more akin to that of the general population, and they did not receive any teaching on this topic during their initial training.

- **Exclusion criteria**

-Unusable questionnaires with less than half the fields completed or illegible.

- Any caregiver who refused to participate in the study.

## 3. Data collection

### 3.1. Data collection tool

In order to achieve our objectives, we developed two questionnaires administered to both populations. The first questionnaire was hetero-administered to the mothers in French (Appendix 1), then translated into Tunisian dialect (Appendix 2). It was an individual questionnaire with closed and open-ended questions. The questionnaire was divided into three parts aimed at determining:

**A. Personal context**

(age, level of education, socio-economic level, marital status, number of children and their respective ages).

**B. Mothers' knowledge**

(definition of asthma, asthma attacks, asthma control in patients, treatment, sources of information, action plan in the event of an asthma attack...)

**C. Mothers' attitudes and practices**

(inhaled treatment administration technique, inhalation chamber maintenance, environmental control).

We tested the questionnaire with a few hospitalized mothers prior to the survey, in order to validate it and detect ambiguous questions or proposals.

The second questionnaire was self-administered to caregivers in French (Appendix 3). It was an individual questionnaire with both closed and open-ended questions. The questionnaire was divided into three parts aimed at determining :

**A. Personal context**

(age, gender, department, seniority in profession and department, previous asthma training).

**B. Caregivers' knowledge**

(definition of asthma, definition of an asthma attack, treatment, sources of information).

**C. Caregivers' attitudes and practices**

### 3.2. Survey process

Our questionnaire was distributed to each caregiver during a one-to-one interview to explain the objectives, obtain consent and ensure that the various items had been properly understood. The questionnaire was then kept by the caregiver, who returned it to us at the end of the morning, or left it in the office of the ward supervisor. We also introduced ourselves to the mothers and obtained their oral consent. Then one of us read the questions in Tunisian dialect, while the other recorded the answers. At the end of the interview, whenever necessary, we corrected any erroneous information and educated the mother in terms of managing an asthmatic child.

### 3.3. Definitions

**Asthma :**

A heterogeneous condition most often characterized by chronic inflammation of the airways. It is defined by the presence of respiratory symptoms such as wheezing, dyspnoea, chest tightness and cough. These symptoms are variable over time and in intensity, with reversible limitation of expiratory flow [5].

**Asthma attacks:**

Short-lasting paroxysmal attacks of respiratory symptoms (dyspnea, wheezing, chest tightness, etc.) that subside spontaneously or with treatment [5].

**Atopy :**

Genetic predisposition to produce IgE antibodies to certain allergens [6].

**Asthma control:** GINA 2021 criteria for asthma symptom control [7].

| **Sur les 4 dernières semaines** | **Contrôlé** (tous les critères présents) | **Partiellement contrôlé** (1-2 critères présents) **ou** **Non contrôlé** (≥3critères présents) |
|---|---|---|
| Symptômes diurnes | ≤2 x/semaine | >2 x/semaine |
| Limitation des activités | Aucune | Toute limitation |
| Symptômes nocturnes | Aucun | Tout symptôme nocturne |
| Traitement de secours | ≤2 x/semaine | >2 x/semaine |

**Technique for administering inhaled treatment: ( APPENDIX 4-5 ) [8].**

Follow these steps

1- Shake inhaler bottle

2- Place the face mask tightly over the nose and mouth or Place the mouthpiece between the teeth and squeeze the lips around it to create a seal if age > 5 years.

3- Metered-dose inhaler canister facing upwards

4- Leave the mask over the child's nose and mouth for about 15sec after delivering the dose from the inhaler.

5- Start with B2 mimetics if prescribed by the doctor

6- Rinse child's face and mouth after inhalation

**Inhalation chamber maintenance: [9-10]**

We recommend cleaning the inhalation chamber before first use and once a week thereafter. The chamber must be disassembled before cleaning. All parts should be washed in lukewarm, mildly soapy water and then air-dried. Do not rinse with clean water or wipe with a cloth. These precautions will keep the plastic chambers electrostatic-free for up to a week.

The rate of change of the inhalation chamber depends on its type. Here are a few examples:

Babyhaler® has a shelf life of 6 months, even with proper cleaning and use. The Vortex® chamber should be discarded and replaced after 60 disinfections. Aerochamber® Plus chambers should be replaced after 12 months. BERG® type chambers can be used for up to three years.

**Environmental control**: [7].

Environmental control is a cornerstone in the therapeutic management of asthma. It's important to take the necessary steps to avoid exacerbating or triggering an asthma attack. These include:

-Avoid contact with feathered/haired animals.

-Avoid strong odors, tree and flower pollens and dust.

-Stop passive smoking

-Change and wash sheets and blankets regularly in hot water and dry them in the sun to eliminate allergens.

-Ventilate rooms and combat humidity.

-Avoid wool carpets and blankets, as they can accumulate dust and dust mites.

Use zippered mite-proof covers for mattresses, comforters and pillows.

**Action plan for an asthma attack at home: ( APPENDIX 6 )** [8]

For mild-to-moderate asthma attacks, start with short-acting bronchodilators (salbutamol) inhaled at a dose of one puff/2kg (maximum 10 puffs). This procedure can be repeated every 20 minutes for the first hour. Oral systemic corticosteroids (prednisolone) at a dose of 1-2 mg/kg for 3-5 days may be combined.

If there is no clinical improvement, or signs of respiratory severity, start with bronchodilators as described above and consult the emergency room.

## 4. Data capture and analysis

Data were manually tabulated and entered using Statistical Package for Social Sciences version 26 for Windows. Results were represented graphically using EXCEL 2007. Frequencies were compared using the chi-square test or Fischer's exact test, and means were compared using Student's t test. Correlations between the various parameters were assessed using Pearson's correlation test. Differences were considered significant when p was less than 0.05.

## 5. Bibliographic research

Bibliographical searches using various keywords relating to the theme under study were carried out on the following sites:

- www.pubmed.com
- www.googlescholar.com

## 6. Ethical considerations

Before beginning data collection, authorizations were obtained from the heads of the departments concerned (Appendix7) . Study objectives and procedures were clearly explained to mothers and caregivers. Participation in the study was then voluntary, based on oral consent. Furthermore, data collection and analysis respected the anonymity of the participants. We declare no conflict of interest.

# RESULTS

## 1. Response rate and flow chart

Fifty questionnaires were distributed to caregivers. We received 40 copies, giving a response rate of 83.3%. Of these, three were illegible and seven incomplete. We therefore analyzed data from 30 copies.

In the Infant Medicine A and CUP departments, 70 mothers were approached, 62 of whom participated fully in the study, giving a response rate of 88.6% (Figure 1).

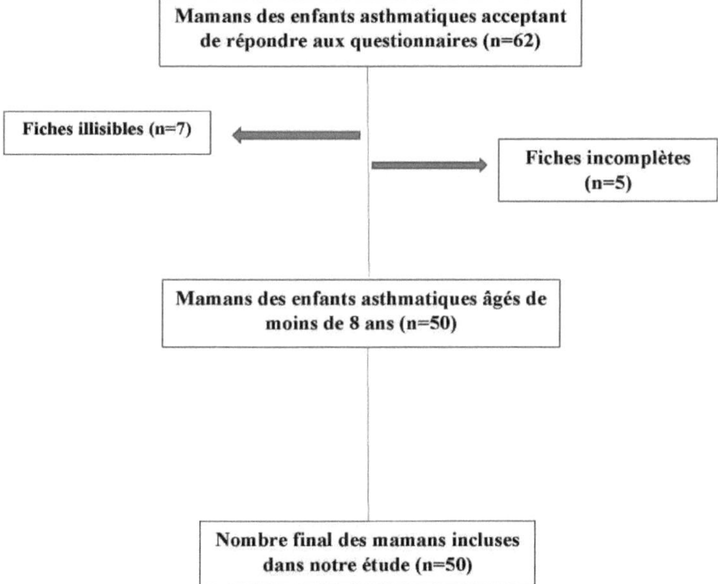


**Figure 1: Diagram of mothers of asthmatic children included in our study**

## 2. Socio-demographic characteristics of study populations

Table I summarizes the socio-demographic characteristics of the mother population. Table II summarizes the socio-demographic data for the caregiver population.

**Table I: Socio-demographic characteristics of the population of asthmatic mothers and children**

| Quantitative variables | N | Average | Min | Max | AND |
|---|---|---|---|---|---|
| Age of mothers (years) | 50 | 37,3 | 20 | 60 | 7,7 |
| Number of years of study (years) | 50 | 10,2 | 2 | 24 | 5,5 |
| Number of dependent children | 50 | 1,5 | 1 | 3 | 1 |

| Qualitative variables | N | Categories | N | % |
|---|---|---|---|---|
| Gender of asthmatic children | 50 | M | 28 | 56 |
| | | F | 22 | 44 |
| Civil status | 50 | Bride | 50 | 100 |
| | | Divorced | 0 | 0 |
| Profession | 50 | Housewife | 47 | 94 |
| | | Civil servant | 3 | 6 |
| Family history of atopy | 25 | Asthma (A) | 22 | 88 |
| | | Allergic rhinitis (R) | 2 | 8 |
| | | (A+R) | 1 | 4 |
| Health education ATCD's about asthma | 50 | YES | 48 | 96 |
| | | NO | 2 | 4 |
| Environmental control | 50 | Humidity | 27 | 54 |
| | | Passive smoking | 31 | 62 |
| | | Feathered and furry animals | 12 | 24 |

%= percentage ; ATCD' s = antecedents ; ET= standard deviation, Max= maximum value of the variable ; Min= minimum value of the variable ; Moy= average value of the variable ; N= total number, n= number by category ; M= male ; F= female

**Table II: Socio-demographic characteristics of the caregiver population**

| Quantitative variables | N | Avg | Min | Max | AND |
|---|---|---|---|---|---|
| Age (years) | 30 | 26 | 20 | 60 | 11,1 |
| Age of diploma (years) | 30 | 8,5 | 1,5 | 25 | 8 |
| Length of service (years) | 30 | 8,8 | 0,1 | 23 | 8 |
| Length of service (years) | 30 | 7,5 | 0,1 | 23 | 7 |

| Qualitative variables | N | Categories | N | % |
|---|---|---|---|---|
| Type | 30 | F | 27 | 90 |
| | | M | 3 | 10 |
| Service | 30 | Ped A | 24 | 80 |
| | | PUC | 6 | 20 |
| Profession | 30 | Nurses | 26 | 86,6 |
| | | Physiotherapist | 2 | 6,7 |
| | | Technician | 2 | 6,7 |
| Initial asthma training | 30 | YES | 14 | 46,7 |
| | | NO | 16 | 53, 3 |
| Asthma continuing education | 30 | YES | 13 | 43,3 |
| | | NO | 17 | 56,7 |
| Care of a child with an asthma attack | 30 | YES | 28 | 93,3 |
| | | NO | 2 | 6,7 |
| Participation in therapeutic education of mothers of asthmatic children | 30 | YES | 6 | 20 |
| | | NO | 24 | 80 |
| Family history of asthma | 30 | YES | 10 | 33,7 |
| | | NO | 20 | 66,7 |

%= percentage; SD= standard deviation, F= female; M= male; Max= maximum value of the variable; Min= minimum value of the variable; Avg= mean value of the variable; N= total number of employees, n= number of employees by category; PEC= care; Péd= paediatric department; PUC= paediatric department, emergencies and consultations.

## 3. Socio-demographic characteristics and control of children asthmatics

We enrolled 50 asthmatic children in our study.

### 3.1. Breakdown by age and gender

The average age of asthmatic children was 4.6±2.3 years, with extremes ranging from 2 to 8 years (Figure 2).

The mean age of the children at diagnosis was 2.8±2 years [0.6- 8 years].

The sex ratio was 1.2.

### 3.2. Associated comorbidity

Among the asthmatic patients, thirteen had gastroesophageal reflux disease and sixteen had allergic rhinitis.

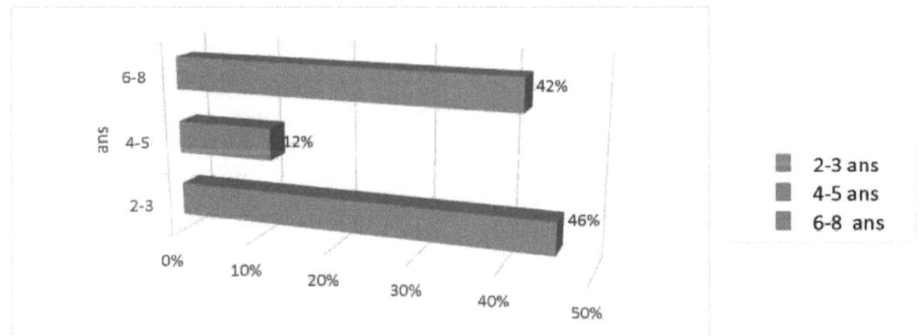


**Figure 2: Age distribution of asthmatic children**

### 3.3. The asthmatic child's environment

Around half the asthmatic children (n=31; 62%) had been exposed to passive smoking and lived in damp homes. Twelve children had pets with feathers or fur.

A minority of patients (n=5) had a single room.

### 3.4. Asthma control and monitoring

#### 3.4.1. Therapeutic compliance

When asked about compliance and the device used, the majority of mothers (n= 37; 74%) had good compliance, and a minority (n= 5; 10%) took inhaled treatment without an inhalation chamber (figure 3).

### 3.4.2. Outpatient follow-up

The majority of patients (n= 30 ;60%) had been followed up regularly at the outpatient clinic every three months, while 12% of patients consulted once a year (figure 4).

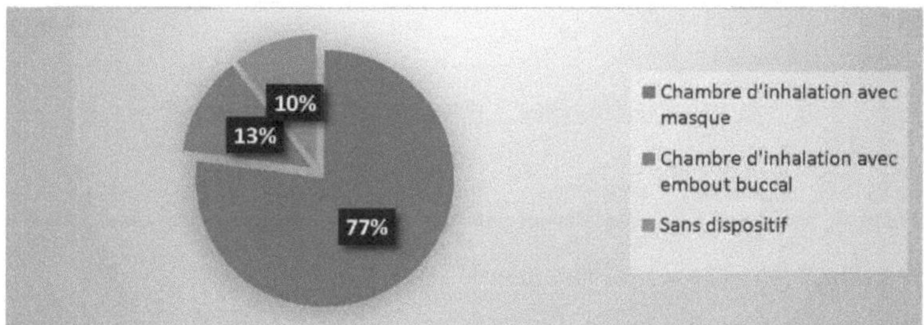


**Figure 3: Device used to take inhaled treatment**

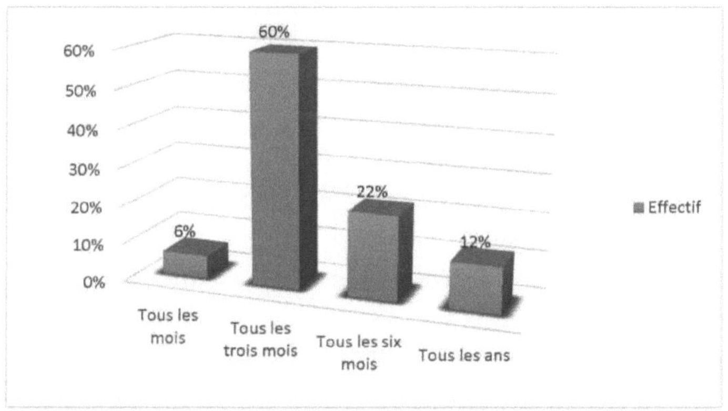


**Figure 4: Follow-up schedule for children with asthma at the outpatient clinic**

### 3.4.3. Number of hospitalizations for asthma attacks in the last year

Around half the patients (n= 23; 46%) had been hospitalized for an asthma attack during the last year of follow-up, 13 of whom were transferred to the intensive care unit (Figure 5). The rate of school absenteeism due to an asthma attack during the last year of follow-up was 28%.

Asthmatic children with poor compliance were the most likely to be hospitalized for asthma attacks (**p= $10^{-3}$** ) and were more likely to be admitted to an intensive care unit (p=10^3 ).

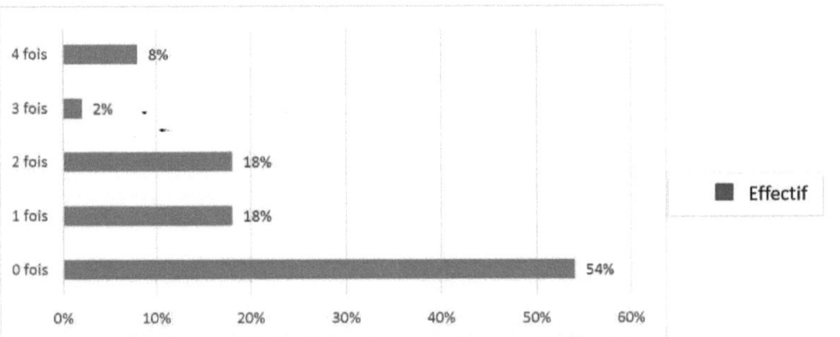


**Figure 5: Number of hospitalizations of asthmatic children during the last year of follow-up**

### 3.4.4 Asthma control over the last month

We assessed our patients' asthma control over the last four weeks according to GINA criteria, and 36% of patients were controlled (daytime symptoms and use of bronchodilators <2 times a week; no nighttime symptoms and no limitation of physical activities).

Nearly half of asthmatic children were partially controlled, while 24% were uncontrolled.

## 4. Knowledge, attitudes and practices of caregivers in the management of asthma in children

### 4.1 Caregivers' knowledge of asthma management in children

Most caregivers (24/30) said they had sufficient knowledge about asthma and its management.

#### 4.1.1. Definition of asthma

Of the 30 caregivers questioned, 60% (n=18) correctly defined asthma as chronic airway inflammation leading to bronchial hyperresponsiveness. The remainder were unable to answer or had given incomplete answers (figure 6).

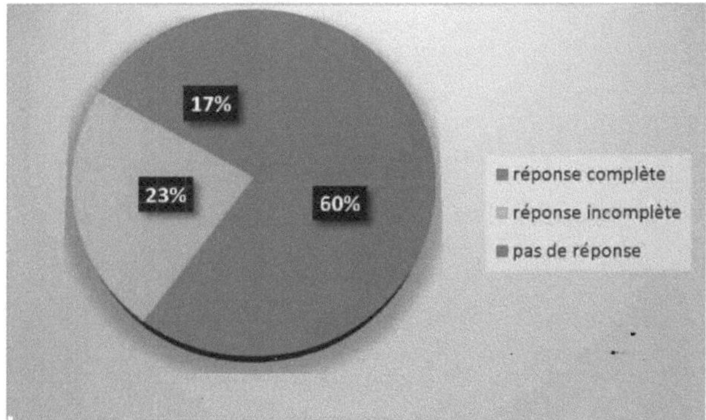


**Figure 6: Caregivers' definition of asthma**

### 4.1.2. Definition of an asthma attack

Of the 30 caregivers questioned, 80% (n=24) correctly defined an asthma attack as a paroxysmal attack of variable and reversible respiratory signs such as wheezing, cough, dyspnea or chest tightness. The others were unable to answer or gave incomplete answers (Figure 7).

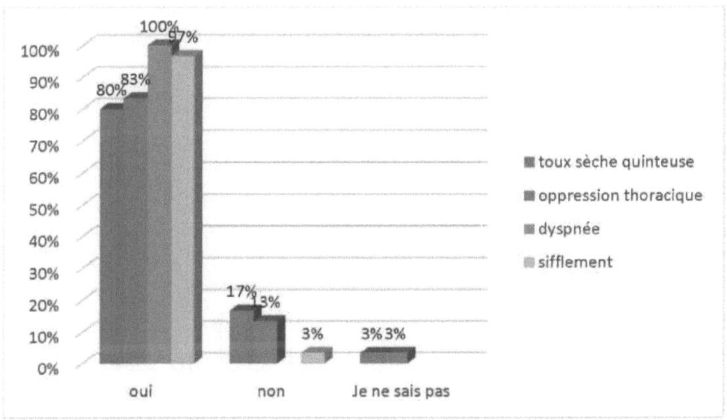


**Figure 7: Definition of asthma attack according to caregivers**

### 4.1.3. Inhaled treatment administration technique :

When asked about the technique and steps involved in administering inhaled treatment, 43% of caregivers (n=13) answered correctly. The remainder gave incomplete answers

(Figure 8).

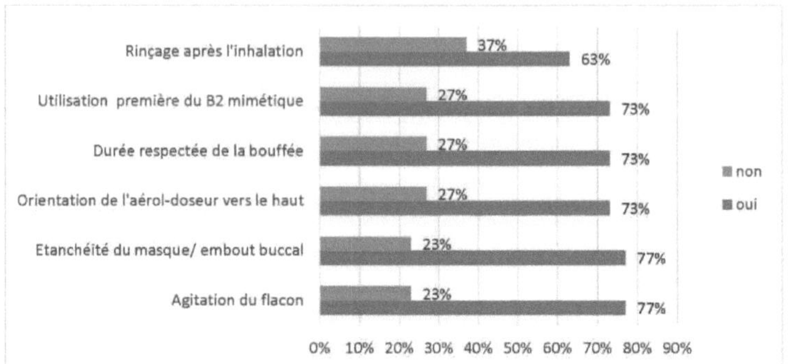


**Figure 8: inhaled treatment administration technique according to caregivers**

### 4.1.4. Inhalation chamber maintenance :

Regarding the frequency of inhalation chamber cleaning, 37% of caregivers (n=11) answered correctly, choosing a weekly frequency. The remainder were unable to answer or gave incorrect answers (Figure 9).

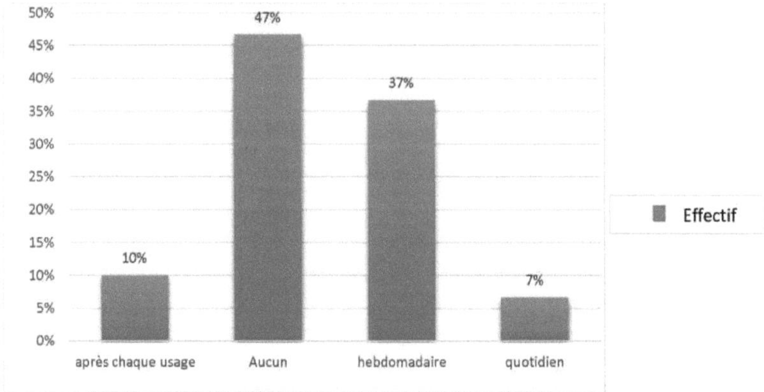


**Figure 9: Inhalation chamber cleaning frequency according to caregivers**

Of the 30 caregivers questioned, around half (n=16; 54%) had answered correctly regarding the product used and the type of water used when cleaning the inhalation chamber. (Figure 10)

The majority of caregivers questioned (n=19; 63%) had also answered correctly concerning the drying of the inhalation chamber, which should be carried out in ambient air, while 17% advocated drying with paper, and the remainder were unable to answer.

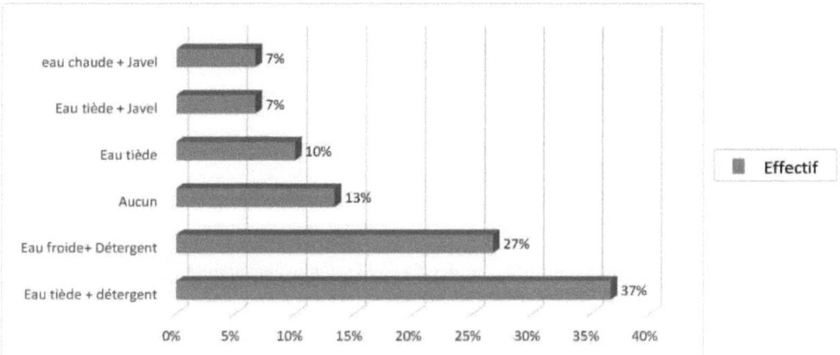


**Figure 10: Type of water and product used to clean the inhalation chamber, according to caregivers**

Nearly half the caregivers (n=14; 46%) had recommended an annual change of inhalation chamber (figure 11).

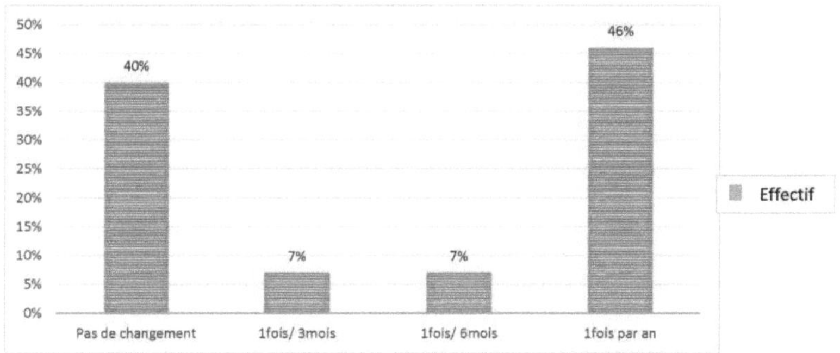


**Figure 11: Rhythm of inhalation chamber change according to caregivers**

### 4.1.5. Environmental control for asthmatic children

A third of the caregivers questioned (n=10; 34%) had given a complete answer concerning the control of the asthmatic child's environment (adequate ventilation of rooms, avoidance of passive smoking, reduction of environmental allergens, maintenance of a clean and hygienic environment...) (Figure 12).

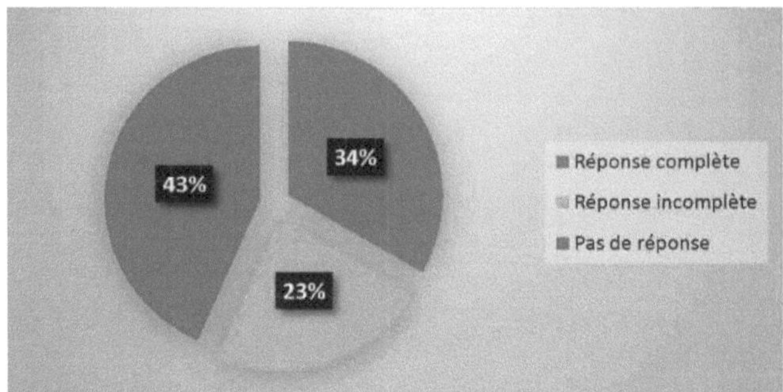


**Figure 12: Control of asthmatic children's environment, according to caregivers**

### 4.2. Caregivers' attitudes and practices in the face of a childhood asthma attack

Around half the caregivers (n=14, 47%) said they were unaware of the principles of asthma attack management, and simply carried out the medical prescription. Seven caregivers gave details of the therapeutic management, while nine caregivers gave incomplete answers (omission of systemic corticosteroid therapy).

### 4.3. Factors associated with caregivers' knowledge, attitudes and practices

**Caregivers' age, department of origin, attendance at initial/continuing asthma education, involvement in asthma education or family history of asthma** did not influence caregivers' knowledge, attitudes or practices.

#### 4.3.1. Influence of seniority in the profession on inhalation chamber maintenance and inhaled treatment administration technique

Knowledge of inhalation chamber maintenance (cleaning product and frequency, drying, etc.) was influenced by seniority in the profession (**$p < 10^{-3}$** ).

We also found a positive correlation between good administration technique and seniority in the profession **(p=0.47; r=0.38).**

### 4.3.2. Influence of seniority in the pediatric ward on asthma definition and inhalation chamber maintenance

We found a negative correlation between the definition of asthma and seniority in the pediatric department **(p=10-3; r= -0.48).** Caregivers recently recruited to the pediatric service defined asthma well.

Knowledge of inhalation chamber maintenance was influenced by seniority in the pediatric department **($p<10^{-3}$ )**.

# 5. Mothers' knowledge, attitudes and practices in the management of childhood asthma

## 5.1. Mothers' knowledge of asthma management in children

Around half the mothers (27/50) said they had sufficient knowledge about asthma and its management. This knowledge came mainly from the medical profession (n=42; 84%) (Figure 13).

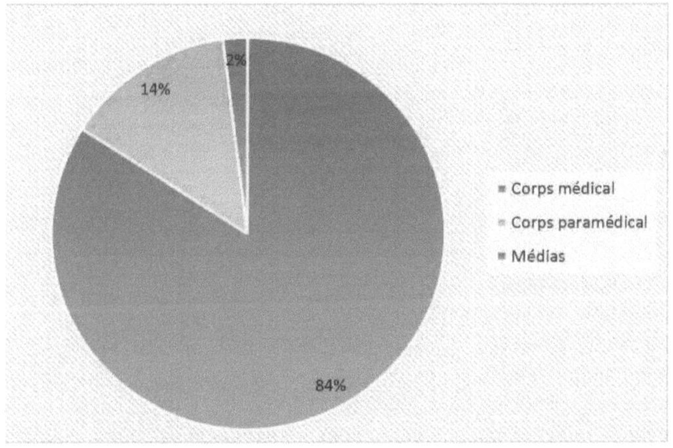


**Figure 13: Mothers' sources of knowledge about asthma management in children**

### 5.1.1. Definition of asthma

Around two-thirds of the mothers (n= 31; 62%) were able to provide some answers regarding the definition of asthma. Ten mothers gave incorrect definitions (asthma is a contagious disease, etc.) (figure 14).

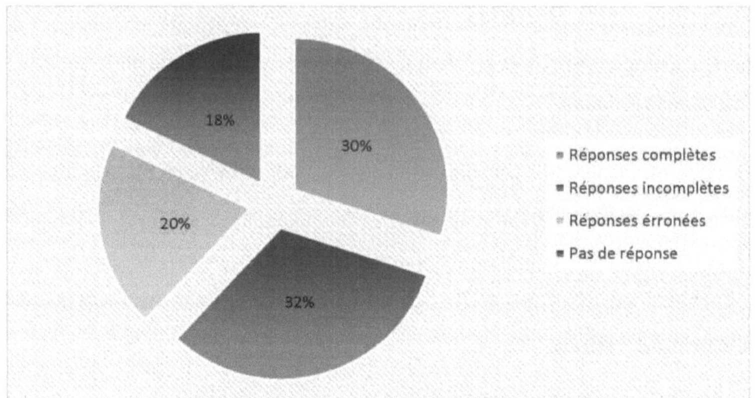


**Figure 14: Mothers' definition of asthma**

### 5.1.2. Definition of an asthma attack

The majority of mothers (n= 44; 88%) were able to provide answers to the question of what constitutes an asthma attack (Figure 15).

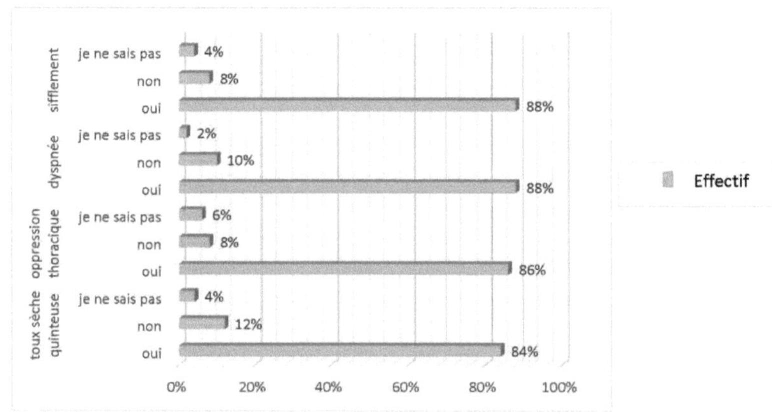


**Figure 15: Definition of asthma attack by mothers**

### 5.1.3. Action plan for asthma attacks

Ten mothers had a correct, well-detailed action plan for an asthma attack.

Half of the mothers (n=25) had omitted an element of therapeutic conduct, such as the time to be respected between puffs of B2 mimetics, or the notion of monitoring for signs of respiratory severity. The remainder consulted the emergency department immediately in the event of an asthma attack, without taking any therapeutic measures at home.

## 5.2.Mothers' attitudes and practices regarding the therapeutic management of asthma

### 5.2.1. Inhaled treatment administration technique :

When asked about the technique and steps involved in administering inhaled treatment, 26% of mothers (n=13) answered correctly. The remainder gave incomplete or incorrect answers (Figure16).

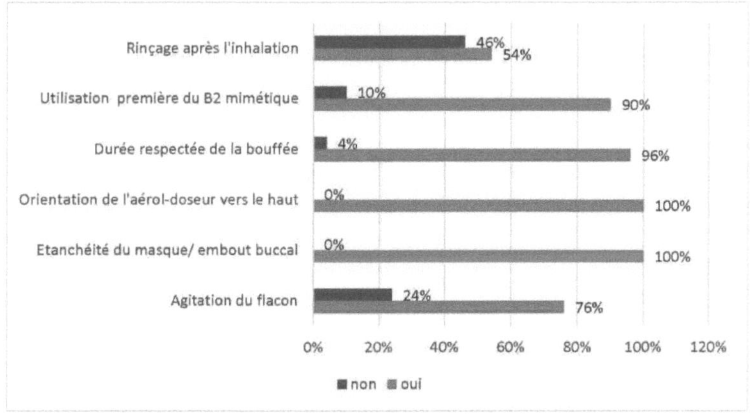


**Figure 16: Technique used by mothers to administer inhaled treatment**

### 5.2.2. Inhalation chamber maintenance :

Around half the mothers (n=30 mothers; 60%) had received education from the nursing staff on how to use and maintain the inhalation chamber. Regarding the frequency of cleaning the inhalation chamber, 26% of mothers (n=52) had answered correctly, choosing a weekly frequency. The remainder were unable to answer or gave incorrect answers (Figure 17).

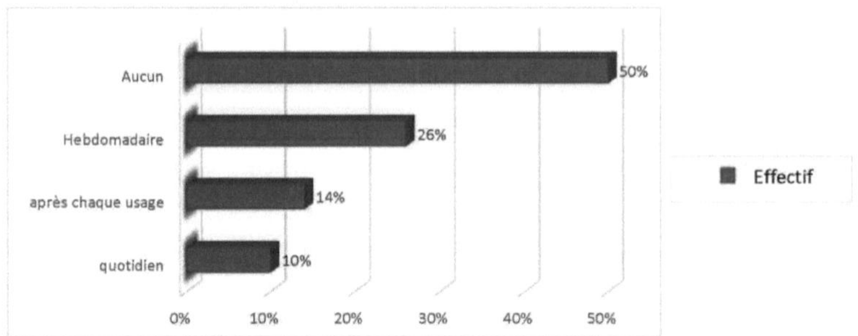


**Figure 17: Inhalation chamber cleaning rhythm according to mothers**

Of the 50 mothers questioned, around half (n=22; 44%) gave correct answers concerning the product used and the type of water used to clean the inhalation chamber. Four mothers gave no answer at all, and the others gave wrong answers.

The majority of the mothers questioned (n=36; 72%) had also answered correctly when it came to drying the inhalation chamber, which should be done with ambient air, while 18% recommended drying with paper, and the remainder had no answer (n=5; 10%).

Nearly half the mothers surveyed (n= 22; 44%) had never changed their inhalation chambers (figure 18).

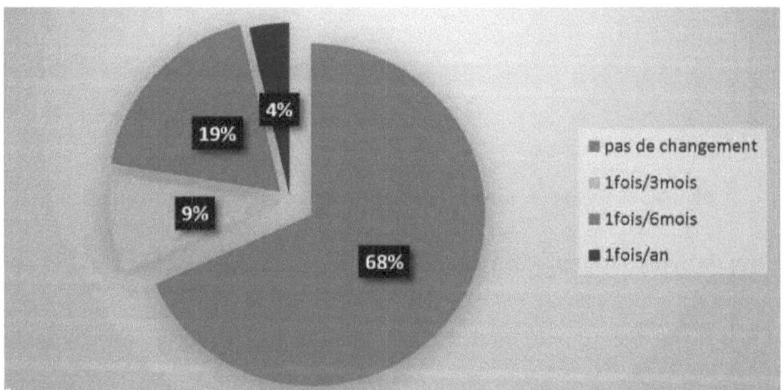


**Figure 18: Pace of inhalation chamber changes according to mothers**

### 5.2.3. Environmental control for asthmatic children

Among the mothers questioned, 26% (n=13) had given a complete answer concerning the control of the asthmatic child's environment (adequate ventilation of rooms, avoidance of passive smoking, reduction of environmental allergens, maintenance of a clean and hygienic environment...) (Figure 19).

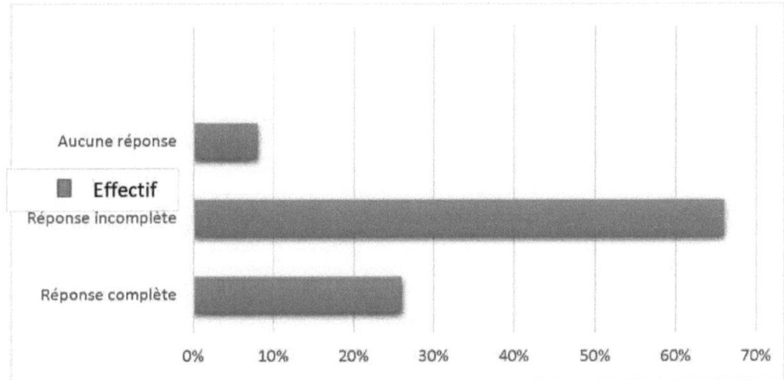


**Figure 19: Control of asthmatic children's environment, according to mothers**

### 5.3. Factors associated with mothers' knowledge, attitudes and practices

**Mothers' age, level of education and profession** did not influence their knowledge, attitudes or practices.

#### 5.3.1. Factors associated with mothers' knowledge

**Source of information**

Physician-educated mothers had a better definition of an asthma attack and a more detailed plan of action in the event of an asthma attack (Table III).

**Table III: Influence of asthma education by the medical profession on mothers' knowledge**

| ASTHMA EDUCATION BY THE MEDICAL PROFESSION | |
|---|---|
| **Mothers' knowledge** | **P** |
| Definition of an asthma attack | **0,034** |
| Action plan for asthma attacks | **0,034** |

### 5.3.2 Factors associated with mothers' attitudes and practices

**Source of information**

The source of information had an influence on inhaler chamber maintenance technique and inhaled treatment administration. Mothers educated by the medical profession had more correct answers (Table IV).

**Table IV: Influence of asthma education by the medical profession on mothers' attitudes and practices**

| ASTHMA EDUCATION BY THE MEDICAL PROFESSION | |
|---|---|
| **Mothers' attitudes and practices** | **P** |
| **Product used to clean the IC** | $10^{-3}$ |
| **Type of water used for CI cleaning** | $10^{-3}$ |
| **IC drying** | $10^{-3}$ |
| **CI cleaning rhythm** | $10^{-3}$ |
| **CI rate of change** | $10^{-3}$ |
| **Technique for administering inhaled therapy** | $10^{-3}$ |

CI: inhalation chamber; ttt: treatment

## History of asthma in siblings

The asthmatic child's environmental control was influenced by the presence of asthma in the siblings **(p=0.04).**

# DISCUSSION

## 1. Study framework and main results

Asthma is the most chronic respiratory disease in the world, with a high morbidity and mortality rate [11] . Management must be early and well adapted to preserve normal respiratory function and guarantee optimal quality of life.

Given that poor adherence to therapy and erroneous practices (poor inhalation technique, defective hygiene of the inhalation chamber, etc.) are the most common factors leading to hospitalization for asthma attacks or exacerbations, and that adherence to treatment in young infants depends on the people around them, education of parents and caregivers has a vital and indisputable role to play in the management of asthmatic children. Both must have a minimum of accurate knowledge to enable them to adjust their practices.

This was the context of our work. Our research question focused on the reasons for mothers' erroneous practices in the therapeutic management of asthma, and the extent to which caregivers were involved. We carried out a descriptive cross-sectional CAP study based on two anonymous questionnaires. One was completed by consenting mothers recruited from the 'A' children's medicine and PUC departments of the Béchir Hamza children's hospital (N=50). The second was completed by physiotherapists, nurses and paediatric technicians working at the Tunis Children's Hospital in the two paediatric departments mentioned above (N=30).

The knowledge and practices of both mothers and caregivers were deemed insufficient.

We found poor compliance in thirteen of our asthma patients. Ten patients received their inhaled treatments without an inhalation chamber, with a poorly controlled environment in 43 cases (passive smoking (n=31), pets (n=12).

Asthma was controlled in 36% of cases. However, during the final year of follow-up, almost half the patients (n=23) were admitted for asthma attacks, 13 of whom were transferred to the intensive care unit.

Asthmatic children with poor compliance were the most likely to be hospitalized for asthma attacks ($p=10^{-3}$ ) and were more likely to be admitted to an intensive care unit ($p=10^{-3}$ ).

Most caregivers were able to put forward the main elements of the definition of asthma and asthma attack. However, almost half the caregivers were unable to describe the main items of inhaled treatment administration technique, maintenance of the inhalation chamber, control of the asthmatic child's environment and behaviour in the event of an asthma attack. Knowledge of inhalation chamber maintenance and inhaler administration technique was influenced by seniority in the profession ($p<10^{-3}$ ) and seniority in the pediatric department ($p<10^{-3}$ ).

The majority of moms were able to put forward some elements of the definition of asthma and asthma attack. Only ten mothers had correctly detailed their action plans in the event of an asthma attack. The source of information: the medical profession was associated with this good knowledge (definition and action plan for an asthma attack) ($p<10^{-3}$ ). Attitudes and practices concerning inhalation chamber maintenance, administration of inhaled treatment and environmental control were controversial. However, almost a third of the mothers had correct practices. Also, physician education ($p<10^{-3}$ ) was associated with good practices. While environmental control ($p=0.04$) was influenced by the presence of asthmatic siblings.

## 2. Study strengths and limitations

### 2.1. Study highlights

The results of this study are very interesting. On the one hand, it is the most frequent chronic respiratory pathology in the world, with a high morbi-mortality rate. On the other hand, this study illustrates how asthma is managed by mothers and caregivers in Tunisia.

### 2.2. Study limitations

Certain biases should be highlighted:

- In our study, mothers and caregivers were selected without prior sampling.
- What's more, the numbers collated may be considered insufficient to assess the knowledge of Tunisian mothers and caregivers as a whole, which reduces their representativeness.
- The hetero-administered nature of the mothers' questionnaire may influence responses.
- A judgment bias, as we collected the answers ourselves (investigator = evaluator).
-

### 2.3. Difficulties encountered

In the course of our investigation we encountered a number of difficulties:

- Mothers were interviewed in a stressful context (during their children's hospitalization, or waiting for their turns at the consultation).
- In a space that is often inappropriate (as it can be heard by others), which can modify and influence their responses.
- Caregivers were also in a hurry because of the workload.

## 3. Comparison of results with the literature :

### 3.1. Response rate

The response rate was high among mothers (88.6%) and caregivers (83.3%), reflecting the importance of the subject.

### 3.2. Definition of asthma and asthma attacks

It's important to know the main definitions of asthma and asthma attacks, so you can adhere to treatment and take the necessary steps in an emergency.

In our study, most caregivers and mothers were able to define asthma and asthma attacks broadly. Several studies have supported our findings, reporting good knowledge on the part of caregivers and mothers [12-14].

The correct definition of an asthma attack, according to our study, was correlated with the education provided by the medical staff ($p=0.034$). Also, a negative correlation was observed between the definition of asthma and seniority in the pediatric department ($p = 10^{-3}$), indicating that recently recruited caregivers had better knowledge.

These results could be explained by the lack of ongoing asthma training among caregivers [15-16].

### 3.3. Compliance with inhaled treatment

In our study, we found poor compliance with treatment in 26% of cases, which increased the risk of hospitalization for asthma attacks ($p<10^{-3}$) and also the risk of an intensive care stay ($p<10^{-3}$).

Indeed, most parents expressed concern about the side effects of inhaled corticosteroids, notably growth retardation, and discontinued treatment without medical advice [17-18].

It is crucial to emphasize to parents that regular monitoring of patients and good compliance with therapy will help preserve near-normal respiratory function, reduce the risk of attacks and subsequently the risk of recurrent hospitalizations, and thus limit the need for additional medication. Appropriate education will lead to better disease management [3-4,19].

### 3.4 Disease monitoring

More than half of our patients (60%) consulted us on a regular basis, with optimal follow-up. To encourage treatment follow-up, it is important to provide clear, targeted explanations of treatment objectives and strategy. It is also important to allow sufficient time for consultations, and to strengthen the doctor-patient relationship.

### 3.5. Technique for administering inhaled treatment and maintenance of the inhalation chamber

In our study, the knowledge, attitudes and practices of caregivers and mothers regarding inhalation chamber maintenance and inhaled therapy administration technique were found to be inadequate. Plaza et al. found that only 15.5% of caregivers gave correct answers concerning the use of inhalation devices, which could subsequently hamper the quality of education for mothers [20]. Hence the importance of reinforcing the training and continuing education of caregivers in order to improve the quality of care offered to asthma patients. Effective inhaled treatment administration techniques also need to be reproduced with mothers, so that errors can be corrected when they occur, and effective medication administration can be guaranteed in the end [21].

#### 3.5.1. The influence of mothers' level of education

We did not find a statistically significant relationship between the educational level of the mothers included in the study and the quality of care provided to their children. However, a descriptive study carried out at the Abderrahmane Mamie Hospital in Tunis showed that parents' level of education had no influence on treatment adherence, inhalation technique or disease follow-up [22]. These data underline the importance of awareness-raising and ongoing education of parents, irrespective of their level of education, for optimal management of this chronic pathology.

#### 3.5.2. Influence of family history of asthma

In our study, almost half of our asthma patients had a family history of asthma, which improved environmental control ($p = 0.04$).

Also, a study conducted at the Béchir Hamza Children's Hospital concluded that the presence of asthma in siblings was statistically associated with mothers' good knowledge and practical attitudes ($p = 0.05$) [23].

#### 3.5.3. Influence of information source

In our study, physician education was statistically associated with good asthma treatment knowledge and practices ($p<10^{-3}$ ). The main source of information was the medical profession (84%). This result has been supported by several studies [318].

This implies the crucial role of physicians in the initial and ongoing training of the paramedical profession, in order to correct erring knowledge, attitudes and practices in asthma management. However, mothers' practices must always be regularly assessed, re-educated at every consultation, and an initial practical demonstration carried out to optimize treatment [20].

### 3.6. Action plan for asthma attacks

A minority of mothers (n=10) were correct in their answers to the question of what to do in the event of an asthma attack. To encourage control of attacks at home and limit the need for emergency care, it is essential to explain treatment to parents, provide a written action plan and, above all, highlight the signs of respiratory severity [19].

### 3.7. Environmental control

The asthmatic child's environment was poorly controlled in the majority of our patients (43/50), 31 of whom lived in damp homes.

There was a lack of knowledge and practice in this area. Indeed, only a third of the mothers gave a complete answer. Despite targeted education, it must be admitted that poor socio-economic conditions can often hinder optimal environmental control [24].

## 4. Recommendations / Role of the childcare licensee :

In order to improve mothers' knowledge and practices, these target mothers need to be offered appropriate health education, by a source suited to this task (well-trained doctors and childcare graduates). We therefore recommend

### 4.1. Nursing staff

- ✓ Attend ongoing training courses and update your knowledge.
- ✓ Manage all asthma exacerbations and attacks.
- ✓ Make parents aware of the importance of treatment to preserve normal respiratory function.
- ✓ Strengthening the caregiver-patient relationship.
- ✓ The childcare graduate could help train his or her colleagues in the treatment of moderate to severe asthma attacks, and educate them on the main therapeutic aspects of asthma.

### 4.2. To mothers:

- ✓ Encourage compliance with treatment to avoid frequent hospitalization for asthma attacks or exacerbations.
- ✓ Raise awareness of inhaled treatment administration techniques and maintenance of the inhalation chamber.
- ✓ Raise awareness of the importance of hygiene measures to control the asthmatic child's environment.
- ✓ Explain the course of action to be taken in the event of an asthma attack at home, or provide a written plan of action.
- ✓ Consult the emergency room if the asthma action plan fails, or if signs of respiratory severity appear.

### 4.3. Health authorities

- ✓ Promote ongoing training in asthma management for nursing staff
- ✓ Provide emergency departments and wards with brochures and posters on inhalation chamber maintenance, inhaler administration techniques and the asthma crisis action plan (appendices 8 ).
- ✓ Educational messages need to be varied, aimed at all mothers, especially those who are homemakers and come from rural areas (impact of audiovisuals via educational spots).

# CONCLUSIONS

Asthma, a heterogeneous, multifactorial pathology caused by chronic inflammation of the bronchi, is the most common chronic respiratory disease in paediatrics. The economic and medical burden of asthma is considerable, with frequent hospitalization and absenteeism from school and work for children and their parents. Therapeutic management is multi-faceted and depends on the child's environment, and is continued if necessary by the caregivers, who must educate and support the parents.

Our research question focused on the reasons for mothers' erroneous practices in the therapeutic management of asthma, and to what extent caregivers intervene.

We carried out a descriptive cross-sectional CAP study based on two anonymous questionnaires. One was completed by consenting mothers recruited from the 'A' children's medicine and PUC departments of the Béchir Hamza children's hospital (N=50). The second was completed by physiotherapists, nurses and paediatric technicians working at the Tunis Children's Hospital in the two paediatric departments mentioned above (N=30). Data were analyzed using Statistique Package for Social Sciences version 26 for Windows. Results were represented graphically using EXCEL 2007. Differences were considered significant when p was less than 0.05.

The response rate was high among both mothers (88.6%) and caregivers (83.3%). We enrolled 50 asthmatic children, with a mean age of 4.6±2.3 years [2-8 years]. The mean age of the children at diagnosis was 2.8±2 years [0.6- 8 years]. The sex ratio was 1.2. Poor compliance was found in thirteen asthmatic patients. Ten patients did not use the inhalation chamber. The asthmatic child's environment was poorly controlled in 43 cases (passive smoking (n=31), pets (n=12)). Asthma was controlled in 36% of cases. Almost half the patients (n=23) were admitted for asthma attacks during the last year of follow-up, 13 of whom were transferred to the intensive care unit. Asthmatic children with poor compliance were more likely to be hospitalized for asthma attacks ($p= 10^{-3}$ ) and more likely to be admitted to an intensive care unit ($p=10^{-3}$ ).

We recruited 50 married mothers, with an average age of 37.3±7.7 years and a median number of 1.5 dependent children. They had previously received health education on the subject in 96% of cases. Around half of the mothers (27/50) claimed to have sufficient knowledge about asthma and its therapeutic management, which came mainly from the medical profession (84%). Around two-thirds of the mothers (n= 31; 62%) were able to give some indication of the definition of asthma, and 88% of them were able to identify the main symptoms of an asthma attack. Only ten moms had a correct and well-detailed plan of action in the event of an asthma attack, while half (n=25) gave incomplete answers. Nearly a third of the mothers (n=13) were able to give the main steps in maintaining the inhalation chamber, the technique for administering inhaled treatment and controlling the asthmatic child's environment. Mothers' age, level of education and occupation had no influence on their knowledge, attitudes or practices.

The source of information: the medical profession ($p<10^{-3}$) was associated with mothers' good knowledge (definition and action plan in the event of an asthma attack) and good practices (treatment administration technique, inhalation chamber maintenance). Environmental control (p=0.04) was influenced by the presence of asthmatic siblings.

We recruited 30 caregivers, most of whom were women (sex ratio 0.11). Average age was 26±11.1 years. The average length of service in the profession and in the paediatric department was 8.8 and 7.5 years respectively. Around half the caregivers (n=14) had received initial/continuing training in asthma and its management. Most of them (24/30) declared that they had sufficient knowledge about asthma. The majority of caregivers (60-80%) knew the main elements of the definition of asthma and the main symptoms of an asthma attack. Nearly half (13/30) were able to detail the technique for administering inhaled treatment. With regard to inhalation chamber maintenance, 19/30 were unable to specify the cleaning schedule, but were able to describe the drying procedure, 16 were able to mention the product used, and 40% were unable to specify the schedule for changing the chamber. One-third of the caregivers questioned (n=10) gave a complete answer concerning environmental control of asthmatic children (adequate ventilation of rooms, avoidance of passive smoking, reduction of environmental allergens, maintenance of a clean and hygienic environment, etc.). 14 caregivers stated that they were not familiar with the principles of asthma attack management, and were content to carry out the medical prescription, while seven out of thirty were able to give details of therapeutic management. Caregivers' age, department of origin, attendance at initial/continuing asthma education courses, involvement in asthma education for children or family history of asthma had no influence on their knowledge, attitudes or practices.

Knowledge of inhalation chamber maintenance and inhaled therapy administration technique was influenced by seniority in the profession ($p<10^{-3}$ ) and seniority in the pediatric department ($p<10^{-3}$ ).

At the end of this study, and given the gaps in knowledge and practices, we recommend..:

- ✓ Promote caregiver education through continuing education sessions.
- ✓ More health education sessions.
- ✓ Use resources adapted to mothers' level of education (leaflets, audio-visual programs to encourage sharing, brochures, website....)

# REFERENCES

1. Gras D, Bourdin A, Chanez P, Vachier I. Bronchial remodeling in asthma: Clinical and respiratory functional consequences. médecine/sciences. nov 2011;27(ll):959-65.

2. Bouayad Z, Afif H. Epidemiology of asthma and rhinitis in southern Mediterranean countries. Rev Fr Allergol. 1998;38(7):155-9.

3. Pointaire D. Enquête d'évaluation des pratiques professionnelles en médecine générale en Martinique en 2015: Prise en charge de l'asthme [thesis: medicine], Antilles: Université des Antilles et de la Guyane; 2015.

4. Carvelli T, Battisti O. How can we practically improve medication compliance in childhood and adolescent asthma? Rev Med Liege.2010;65(5):343-9.

5. FitzGerald JM, Reddel H, Boulet LP. Pocket guide to asthma treatment and prevention. [Online]. Feb 2016 [accessed March 8, 2024]; [32 pages]. Available from URL: https://ginasthma.org/wp-content/uploads/2016/09/WMS-French-Pocket-Guide-GINA- 2016.pdf

6. Oettgen HC, Geha RS. IgE regulation and roles in asthma pathogenesis. J Allergy Clin Immunol. March 1, 2001;107(3):429-41.

7. Reddel HK, Bacharier LB, Bateman ED, Brightling CE, Brusselle GG, Buhl R, et al. Global Initiative for Asthma Strategy 2021: Executive Summary and Rationale for Key Changes. Am J Respir Crit Care Med. Ijanv 2022;205(l):17-35.

8. Mauer Y, Taliercio RM. Managing adult asthma: The 2019 GINA guidelines. Cleve ClinJMed. August 31, 2020;87(9):569-75.

9. VIDAL. How to maintain an inhalation chamber? [Online]. Oct 2013 [accessed March 8, 2024]; [37 pages]. Available from URL:

10. Nault D, Battisti L, Beauchesne MF, Bouchard J, Boulet LP, Dagenais J, et al. Techniques and maintenance of inhalation devices. [Online]. Oct 2019 [Accessed March 8, 2024]. Available from URL: https://www.vidal.fr/medicaments/utilisation/medicaments- children/using-chamber-inhalation-children.html

11. Demoly P, Godard P, Bousquet J. An overview of asthma epidemiology. Rev Fr Allergol Immunol Clin. 1 Oct 2005;45(6):464-75.

12. Evaluation of the knowledge and practices of health professionals on the

diagnosis of childhood asthma in Niamey. J Funct Vent Pulmonol. 30 Nov 2016;7(22):40-5.

13. Belloumi N, Bougacha M, Habouria C, Bachouche I, Chermiti Ben Abdallah F, Fenniche S. Level of knowledge about occupational asthma and asthmogenic agents: evaluation among healthcare personnel using a validated questionnaire. Rev Mal Respir. Oct 1, 2023;40(8):655-65.

14. Bemba ELP, Adambounou TAS, Koumeka PP, Bopaka RG, Ossale Abacka KB, Mboussa J. Evaluation of knowledge and practices on the management of asthma in rural Congo. Rev Fr Allergol. Oct 1, 2019;59(6):440-6.

15. Haouichat H, Benali R, Benyounes A, Berrabah Y, Douagui H, Guermaz M, et al. Asthma control in adults in Algeria. Comparison with other North African and Middle Eastern countries. Rev Mal Respir. 2020;37(1):15-25.

16. Masson E. EM-Consulte. [cited May 7, 2024]. Mortality in asthma in Africa: about 35 cases collected in the three CHU of Abidjan, Ivory Coast. Available at: https://www.em-consulte.com/article/196602/mortalite-dans-lasthme-en-afriquec-a-propos- de-35c

17. Caseaux A. Evaluation of the perception of inhaled corticosteroids among parents of asthmatic children aged 4 to 10 years in Lorraine: a quantitative study using a validated questionnaire [Internet][other]. Université de Lorraine; 2017 [cited 2024 May 5]. p. Not provided. Available from: https://hal.univ-lorraine.fr/hal-01932115

18. Zhao J, Shen K, Xiang L, Zhang G, Xie M, Bai J, et al. The knowledge, attitudes and practices of parents of children with asthma in 29 cities of China: a multi-center study. BMC Pediatr. Feb 4, 2013;13(1):20.

19. Rougeot K. État des connaissances des parents d'enfants asthmatiques sur la maladie asthmatique et sa prise en charge, dans le Sud de la Réunion entre 2016 et 2017 [thesis: medicine]. Bordeaux: Université de Bordeaux; 2019.

20. Plaza V, Giner J, Rodrigo GJ, Dolovich MB, Sanchis J. Errors in the Use of Inhalers by Health Care Professionals: A Systematic Review. J Allergy Clin Immunol Pract. May 1, 2018;6(3):987-95.

21. Gillette C, Rockich-Winston N, Kuhn JA, Flesher S, Shepherd M. Inhaler Technique in Children With Asthma: A Systematic Review. Acad Pediatr. 2016;16(7):605-15.

22. M'Barek NEH, Khalfallah I, Hamdi B, Smaoui R, Ammar J, Hamzaoui A. Impact of parents' education level in the evolution of childhood asthma. Rev Mal Respir Actual. 1 Jan 2020;12(1):187.

23. Khalsi F, Mansouri H, Briki I, Kbaier S, Trabelsi I, Belhadj I, et al. Knowledge and perceptions of parents of asthmatic children. Rev Fr Allergol. 1 Apr 2023;63(3):103569.

24. Kamps AWA, Brand PLP, Roorda RJ. Determinants of correct inhalation technique in children attending a hospital-based asthma clinic. Acta Paediatr Oslo Nor 1992. 2002;91(2):159-63.

25. Asthma | National College of University Pediatricians - www.pedia-univ.fr [Internet]. [cited May 24, 2024]. Available from: https://www.pedia-univ.fr/deuxieme-cycle/referentiel/pneumologie-cardiologie/asthme .

26. CHU Sainte-Justine : hôpital mère enfant de Montréal [Internet], [cited May 24 2024]. Available from: https://www.chusj.org/.

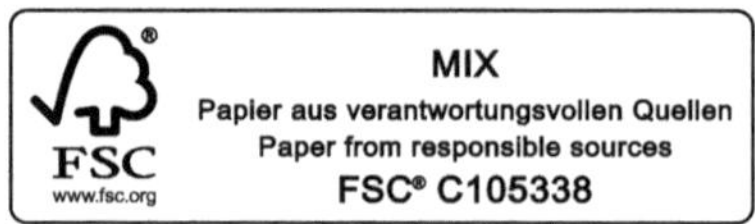


Printed by Books on Demand GmbH, Norderstedt / Germany